Low Carb

Trying To Cut Back On Carbs?

Top 45 Low Carb Recipes That Help You Lose Weight While Still Enjoying Delicious Food

Table Of Contents

Introduction

Do you want to get started on a low carb diet right now? Let this recipe book help you out! Learn the top 45 delicious and easy to prepare low carb dishes from around the world.

There are many ways to make your low carb diet more interesting. Add variety in flavor and nutritional content to your everyday meals by choosing from these carefully designed recipes.

In this book you will find breakfast recipes, including low carb muffins and waffles (did you know that these are even possible?), snacks that even your friends will enjoy, soups, poultry, beef, pork, hot vegetable, and seafood recipes for your lunch and dinner meals. You will also find delectable desserts that will satisfy your sweet tooth without the extra carb!

Get creative in the kitchen and start whipping up these delicious low carb recipes. Making your meal plans will be a lot more fun once you have got so many flavors to choose from.

Thanks again for buying this book, I hope you enjoy it!

Chapter 1 - Getting Started on Low Carb

If you really want to lose weight and jumpstart a healthier lifestyle, one highly recommended step is to cut down the carbohydrates in your diet. Many people from all over the world experience amazing results in both their outward appearances and how they feel (including their energy levels) once they have learned to control their carb intake.

Carbohydrates are responsible for increasing blood sugar, which then increases insulin levels. The simple carbs such as those in white flour, white rice, pasta, and sugar are the unhealthiest. They are mostly responsible for the weight gain, heart disease, and high blood pressure that many individuals suffer from nowadays.

The low carb diet is not just for those who want to lose weight. People who have insulin resistance and are at risk for developing type 2 diabetes should also talk to their doctors regarding this type of diet.

Of course, just because you are planning on cutting carbs does not mean you will no longer enjoy delicious food. On the contrary, you will still be able to savor a wide range of flavors even without having to eat carb on a regular basis. There are so many fruits, vegetables, meats, seafood, poultry, and other food products to choose from and add to your meal plans. You can even use alternatives to wheat flour in making muffins, cakes, cookies and other baked goods. This recipe will share with you a wide range of yummy choices to choose from.

Chapter 2 - Breakfast

Protein Waffles

Makes: 5 servings

Ingredients:

- 1/4 cup raw wheat germ
- 1/4 cup vanilla-flavored whey protein powder
- 1/2 cup soy powder
- 1/4 tsp salt
- 1/2 Tbsp Splenda
- 1/4 cup sesame seeds
- 2 eggs
- 1/3 cup heavy cream
- 1/4 cup water
- 3 Tbsp melted butter

Instructions:

1. Preheat your waffle iron.

2. In a mixing bowl, combine the soy powder, whey protein powder, wheat germ, sesame seeds, salt, and Splenda.

3. Separate the egg and set aside the yolks in a bowl. Beat the whites until they are stiff, and then set aside.

4. Add the water, oil, and cream to the yolks and whisk to combine. Pour the yolk mixture into the powder mixture and combine well. Carefully fold in the egg whites.

5. Ladle some of the batter onto the waffle iron and bake until golden brown. Repeat until you have used up all of your batter. Serve with sugar-free jelly, syrup, butter, cinnamon, and/or fresh berries.

Chorizo Frittata

Makes: 2 servings

Ingredients:

- 1/2 Tbsp oil

- 1/2 small onion, sliced

- 1/4 green bell pepper, diced

- 1/6 cup cooked, crumbled, and drained chorizo

- 1/6 cup salsa

- 4 eggs, beaten

- 3 oz shredded Monterey Jack or Cheddar cheese

Instructions:

1. Place a heavy-duty skillet over medium flame and heat the oil. Sauté the onion and bell pepper until fork-tender. Add the chorizo and salsa and stir until cooked.

2. Spread out the mixture to create an even layer then place the beaten eggs on top.

3. Decrease the heat to low and cover the skillet with a lid or some aluminum foil. Cook for 6 minutes or until eggs become set.

4. Sprinkle the shredded cheese on top and then place the skillet under the broiler at about 4 inches away from the heat. Broil for 2

minutes or until eggs are set and cheese becomes melted. Slice into wedges, and then serve.

English Muffins

Makes: 6 servings

Ingredients:

- 1/4 cup yogurt
- 1/4 cup warm water
- 1/2 tsp salt
- 1/3 cup vital wheat gluten
- 1/8 cup psyllium husks
- 1 Tbsp raw wheat germ
- 1/8 cup wheat bran
- 1/4 cup oat flour
- 1/4 cup vanilla-flavored whey protein powder
- 3/4 tsp yeast

Instructions:

1. Combine the ingredients following the sequence given and process the machine until you have reached the end of the "rise" cycle. Take out the dough.

2. Sprinkle some oat flour on your work surface to prevent the dough from sticking to it. Pat out the dough until it is approximately half an inch thick.

3. Cut out roughs from the dough using a round cutter the size of a medium-sized tin can or you can also use tin can with the ends removed. Once cut out, cover the pieces with a clean dish cloth and set them aside in a spot with warm temperature to rise for approximately an hour.

4. Place a heavy skillet over medium-low flame and lightly scatter some wheat germ on top to prevent the muffin dough from sticking to it. Put the muffin dough rounds in the skillet and bake for 6 minutes per side or until golden brown.

5. Serve the way you would as regular muffins, with butter, eggs, and/or bacon.

Ham and Cheese Puff

Makes: 2 servings

Ingredients:

- 1/8 lb ham

- 1/8 lb Cheddar cheese

- 2 oz mushrooms, well drained

- 1/2 green bell pepper

- 3 eggs

- 1 1/2 Tbsp soy powder or unflavored protein powder

- 1/4 tsp salt

- 1/4 tsp baking powder

- 1/2 cup small-curd cottage cheese

- 1 Tbsp grated horseradish

Instructions:

1. Preheat the oven to 350 degrees F. Grease a 3 cup casserole with butter or nonstick cooking spray.

2. Attach the S blade to the food processor and finely chop the Cheddar, ham, green bell pepper, and mushrooms together.

3. In a bowl, beat the eggs and combine with the soy or protein powder, salt, and baking

powder. Add the horseradish and cottage cheese and beat well. Add the ham mixture and beat well.

4. Transfer the egg and ham mixture into the prepared casserole and bake for 30 minutes or until puffy but not firm. Slice and serve.

Sour Cream Cinnamon Cake

Makes: 6 slices

Ingredients:

- 1/2 cup sour cream
- 1/4 cup water
- 1/3 cup oil
- 2 eggs
- 1 tsp almond extract
- 1/2 cup and 2 Tbsp vanilla-flavored whey protein powder
- 1/8 cup oat flour
- 1 Tbsp vital wheat gluten
- 1/2 Tbsp baking powder
- 1/2 tsp baking soda
- 1 tsp cinnamon
- 1/4 cup Splenda
- 1/2 Tbsp liquid saccharine sweetener

For the topping:

- 1/4 cup chopped walnuts
- 1/8 tsp cinnamon
- 1 Tbsp Splenda

Instructions:

1. Preheat the oven to 350 degrees F. Grease a spring form pan using nonstick cooking spray or butter.

2. In a bowl, mix together the eggs, sour cream, oil, water, and almond extract until very well blended. Gradually stir in the protein powder, vital wheat gluten, oat flour, baking powder, baking soda, Splenda, cinnamon, and liquid saccharine. Mix well, then transfer into the prepared spring form pan.

3. In a bowl, mix together the ingredients for the toppings and then sprinkle this on top of the batter. Bake for 30 minutes. Take it out of the oven, run a knife along the edges, set aside to cook for a bit, then cut and serve.

Chapter 3 - Snacks

Spinach Stuffed Mushrooms

Makes: 20 pieces

Ingredients:

- 3/4 lb mushrooms, patted dry
- 1/4 cup chopped onion
- 1 Tbsp butter
- 2 cloves garlic, crushed
- 2 oz cream cheese
- 5 oz frozen chopped spinach, thawed
- 1/8 tsp pepper
- 1/4 tsp salt
- 3/4 tsp Worcestershire sauce
- 1/8 cup Parmesan cheese

Instructions:

1. Preheat the oven to 350 degrees F.

2. Chop the stems off the mushrooms and dice them. Set the caps aside.

3. Place a heavy-duty skillet over medium-low flame and melt the butter. Sauté the diced

mushroom stems and the onion until mushroom changes color and onion becomes translucent. Add the garlic and sauté for 2 minutes or until garlic becomes fragrant.

4. Place the spinach into a colander and press as much of the water out as possible. Add the spinach into the mushroom and onion mixture and stir to combine. Add the cream cheese and stir until melted, then add the Worcestershire sauce and Parmesan cheese. Season with salt and pepper.

5. Spoon the cooked spinach and mushroom mixture into the mushroom caps and arrange them on a baking pan. Sprinkle some more Parmesan cheese on top and add a bit of water to cover the base of the pan.

6. Bake for 25 to 30 minutes, then serve.

Low Carb Nachos

Makes: 4 servings

Ingredients:

- 1/2 lb lean ground beef

- 7 1/2 oz canned black soy beans, drained

- 4 oz canned Mexican Hot Style tomato sauce or tomato sauce with 1 1/2 Tbsp enchilada sauce

- 6 oz soy and flaxseed tortilla chips

- 1 cup grated cheese of your choice

- 1 small tomato, diced

- 1/4 cup sliced olives

- Sour cream

Instructions:

1. Place a heavy-duty skillet over medium flame and cook the ground beef until brown and crumbled. Drain the fat and add the black soy beans and tomato sauce. Cook for 2 minutes and stir frequently.

2. Arrange the tortilla chips on a platter and sprinkle half a cup of grated cheese on top. Add the meat and soy bean mixture on top, and then add the remaining cheese. Arrange some olives on top.

3. Microwave the nacho mixture for 30 seconds on high or until cheese melts. Sprinkle the diced tomato and spoon sour cream on top. Serve.

Spinach Balls with Coconut Ginger Sauce

Makes: 4 servings

Ingredients:

- 10 oz frozen chopped spinach, defrosted and dried
- 1 cup almond meal
- 3/4 cup chopped macadamia nuts
- 1/8 tsp garlic powder
- 1/2 tsp salt
- 1 Tbsp dried minced onion
- 1/4 cup Parmesan cheese, grated
- 2 egg whites or 1 egg
- 1/2 stick butter, melted

For the Coconut Ginger Sauce:

- 7 oz coconut milk
- 1/8 tsp garlic powder
- 1/2 Tbsp dried minced onion
- 1/2 Tbsp ground ginger
- 1/6 cup coconut oil

Instructions:

1. Preheat oven to 350 degrees F.

2. Make the coconut ginger sauce by mixing all of the ingredients for it in a bowl.

3. Combine all of the ingredients for the spinach balls in a mixing bowl. With clean hands, form them into 1 inch sized balls. Line them on a greased baking sheet. Pour the coconut ginger sauce all over them.

4. Bake for 15 to 20 minutes. Set aside to cool for a bit, then serve.

Pizza Muffins

Makes: 15 pizza muffins

Ingredients:

- 1 Tbsp olive oil
- 1/4 cup chopped green bell pepper
- 1/4 cup chopped red bell pepper
- 1/4 small onion, chopped
- 1 small clove garlic, minced
- 1/2 cup chopped mushrooms
- 1/8 cup chopped olives
- 1/4 tsp red pepper flakes
- 1 egg
- 1/4 tsp Italian seasoning
- 3/4 cup shredded mozzarella
- 2 Tbsp grated Parmesan cheese
- 4 oz cream cheese, softened
- 15 sliced deli-sized pepperoni
- 1/4 cup sugarless pizza sauce
- Freshly ground black pepper

Instructions:

1. Place a skillet over medium flame and add the olive oil. Sauté the garlic, onion, and bell peppers until soft, then add the mushrooms and sauté for 1 minute. Remove from the heat and add the olives, Italian seasoning, red pepper flakes, and a dash of black pepper.

2. In a small bowl, beat the egg lightly and combine the mozzarella, Parmesan, and cream cheese in it. add the mushroom and olive mixture into it and stir well until thoroughly combined.

3. Prepare some mini-muffin cups and line each with a pepperoni slice to create a "cup". Use a teaspoon to spoon some of the vegetable and cheese mix into each cup.

4. Bake for 15 minutes at 325 degrees F or until lightly browned. Take them out of the oven, add some pizza sauce on top of each, and pop them back in. Bake for an additional 10 minutes.

5. Set aside to cool for 5 minutes, then serve.

Chinese Sticky Wings

Makes: 14 pieces

Ingredients:

- 1 1/2 lb chicken wings

- 1/8 cup soy sauce

- 1/8 cup dry sherry

- 1/8 cup sugar-free imitation honey or maple syrup

- 1 small clove garlic

- 1/2 Tbsp grated ginger root

- 1/4 tsp chili garlic paste

Instructions:

1. Cut the wings into drummettes and put them into a resealable plastic bag.

2. In a bowl, combine all of the other ingredients, then pour this into the plastic bag. Close the bag, making sure to get as much of the air out as possible. Turn the bag several times to coat the chicken wings with the marinade. Refrigerate for 12 to 24 hours.

3. Preheat the oven to 375 degrees F.

4. Take the bag out of the fridge and squeeze the marinade out and into a bowl. Place the wings in a single layer in a shallow baking pan.

5. Bake for 1 hour, basting once every 15 minutes using the marinade. Set aside to cool for a bit, and then serve.

Chapter 4 - Soups

Artichoke Soup

Makes: 3 servings

Ingredients:

- 2 Tbsp butter
- 1 stalk celery, finely chopped
- 1/2 small onion, finely chopped
- 1 small clove garlic, crushed
- 7 oz quartered artichoke hearts, drained
- 2 cups chicken stock
- 1/4 tsp xanthan or guar
- 1/2 cup half-and-half
- 1/4 lemon, juiced
- Salt
- Pepper

Instructions:

1. Place a heavy-duty skillet over medium-low flame and melt the butter. Saute the celery, garlic, and onion.

2. Drain the artichoke hearts and cut off the tough bits of leaf. Put the hearts into a food processor with the S blade attached and pour in 1/4 cup of chicken soup and the xanthan or guar. Puree.

3. Transfer the artichoke mixture into a saucepan and add the rest of the chicken stock. Increase heat to medium-high and let simmer.

4. Once the celery and onion have become tender, add them into the artichoke mixture and stir. Bring to a simmer, then stir in the half-and-half. Let simmer, then add the lemon juice and stir.

5. Season to taste with salt and pepper. Serve hot or chilled.

Mulligatawny

Makes: 3 servings

Ingredients:

- 1 qt chicken broth
- 1 1/4 cup cooked boneless, skinless chicken, iced
- 1 1/2 Tbsp butter
- 1 small clove garlic, crushed
- 1 small onion, chopped
- 1 rib celery, diced
- 1/2 small carrot, shredded
- 1 tsp curry powder
- 1/2 bay leaf
- 1/4 tart apple, finely chopped
- 1/4 tsp pepper
- 1/4 tsp dried thyme
- 1/2 tsp salt
- 1/2 lemon rind, grated
- 1/2 cup heavy cream

Instructions:

1. Pour the broth into a stockpot and add the chicken. Place over low flame.

2. In a heavy-duty skillet, melt the butter and saute the garlic, onion, celery, carrot, and curry powder, until vegetables become soft. Add everything into the stockpot.

3. Put the apple, bay leaf, thyme, lemon, salt, and pepper into the stockpot and let simmer for 30 minutes. Stir in the cream, then serve.

Jamaican Pepper pot Soup

Makes: 3 servings

Ingredients:

- 1 lb boneless beef round or chuck, chopped into 1-inch cubes
- 1/4 lb bacon, diced
- 1 small onion, chopped
- 2 cups water
- 1/2 cup canned beef broth
- 10 oz frozen chopped spinach
- 1/4 tsp dried thyme
- 7 oz sliced tomatoes
- 1/2 green bell pepper, diced
- 1/2 bay leaf
- 1/2 tsp hot sauce
- 1 tsp salt
- 1/4 tsp pepper
- 5 oz sliced okra
- 1 1/2 Tbsp butter
- 1/4 cup heavy cream
- Paprika

Instructions:

1. Combine the beef cubes, bacon, onion, beef broth, and water in a soup pot. Place over medium heat and bring to a boil, then put the heat on low and let simmer for 45 minutes.

2. Add the thyme, green bell pepper, spinach, tomatoes, bay leaf, hot sauce, salt, and pepper. Simmer for an additional 20 minutes.

3. In a skillet over the lowest heat possible, melt the butter and saute the okra for approximately 5 minutes. Scrape the okra and butter into the stockpot and let simmer for 6 to 8 minutes more.

4. Take the stockpot off the flame and stir the cream into the soup. Add a dash of paprika on top and serve.

Turkey Meatball Soup

Makes: 2 servings

Ingredients:

- 1/4 lb ground turkey
- 3/4 Tbsp oat bran
- 1/4 tsp salt
- 1/4 tsp poultry seasoning
- 1/16 tsp pepper
- 1/2 Tbsp olive oil
- 1 Tbsp minced fresh parsley
- 1/4 cup grated carrot
- 1 cup diced zucchini
- 1/2 Tbsp minced onion
- 1/2 qt chicken broth
- 1 small clove garlic, crushed
- 1/2 tsp dried oregano
- 1 egg, beaten
- 1/8 cup grated Parmesan cheese

Instructions:

1. In a large bowl, combine the ground turkey, parsley, 1/4 teaspoon salt, pepper, poultry

seasoning, oat bran, and parsley. With clean hands, mix well then shape into 1-inch balls and set aside.

2. Place a heavy-duty saucepan over medium-high flame and heat the olive oil. Sauté the carrot for 2 minutes, then add the onion, garlic, and zucchini. Sauté for 5 minutes.

3. Pour the chicken broth into the saucepan and add the oregano. Bring to a simmer for 12 minutes, then add the turkey meatballs, one at a time, as you let the soup simmer for 15 minutes.

4. Before serving, pour the beaten egg into the soup and stir slowly to distribute. Simmer for 1 minute, then ladle into soup bowls. Sprinkle with Parmesan cheese on top, then serve.

Low Carb Clam Chowder

Makes: 2 servings

Ingredients:

- 1/4 cup finely chopped onion
- 1/4 cup finely chopped celery
- 4 bacon strips
- 6 1/2 oz canned clams, juices reserved
- 1/2 cup chicken broth
- 1 large turnip, peeled and cut into small cubes
- 1/4 tsp dried thyme
- 1/4 tsp pepper
- Salt
- 1/2 cup heavy cream

Instructions:

1. In a skillet over medium flame, fry the bacon and set aside. Saute the onion and celery in the bacon grease until soft, then remove the vegetables from the skillet and set aside.

2. Using the same skillet, pour in the chicken broth, clam juice, turnip, thyme, salt, and pepper. Cover and cook for about 10 minutes, stirring occasionally, until turnips become fork-tender.

3. Take the skillet off the heat and add the clams and heavy cream. Stir to combine, then crumble the bacon on top. Place over the lowest flame setting to heat through, then serve.

Chapter 5 - Poultry

Spicy Peanut Chicken

Makes: 2 servings

Ingredients:

- 1/2 tsp ground cinnamon

- 1/2 tsp ground cumin

- 2 boneless, skinless chicken breasts

- 1 1/2 Tbsp peanut oil

- 1/2 small onion, sliced thinly

- 8 oz canned diced tomatoes

- 1 Tbsp natural peanut butter

- 1 clove garlic, crushed

- 1/2 Tbsp lemon juice

- 1/2 fresh jalapeno, seeded

Instructions:

1. Combine the cumin and cinnamon in a saucer and rub all over the chicken breasts.

2. Place a heavy skillet over medium flame and heat 1 1/2 tablespoons of the oil. Add the sliced onion and chicken and cook the chicken until browned on both sides.

3. Pour the liquid from the canned diced tomatoes and half of the tomatoes into a food processor and blender. Add the lemon juice, garlic, jalapeno, and peanut butter. Blend until smooth.

4. Pour the peanut butter sauce on top of the chicken in the skillet. Add the remaining canned tomatoes, then cover and reduce heat. Simmer for 10 minutes or until chicken is completely cooked. Serve.

Easy Turkey Loaf

Makes: 2 to 3 servings

Ingredients:

- 1/2 lb ground turkey

- 1/2 rib celery, finely chopped

- 1/2 small onion, finely chopped

- 1/4 cup finely chopped apple

- 1/4 cup crushed pork rinds

- 3/4 Tbsp Worcestershire sauce

- 1 tsp poultry seasoning

- 1/2 tsp salt

- 1 small egg

Instructions:

1. Preheat the oven to 350 degrees F. Grease a loaf pan with oil or nonstick cooking spray.

2. In a large bowl, mix together all of the ingredients by hand until completely combined. Pack the mixture into the prepared loaf pan and bake for 50 minutes.

3. Take it out and run a knife around the edges to loosen the turkey loaf from the pan. Flip and slice. Serve.

Moroccan Stewed Chicken

Makes: 2 to 3 servings

Ingredients:

- 2 lb chicken pieces
- 1/8 cup olive oil
- 1 small onion, sliced thinly
- 1 clove garlic, crushed
- 1/3 cup chicken broth
- 1/4 tsp ground cinnamon
- 1/4 tsp ground coriander
- 1/4 tsp paprika
- 1/4 tsp ground cumin
- 1/2 tsp ground ginger
- 1/4 tsp pepper
- 1/8 tsp cayenne
- 1/2 Tbsp Splenda
- 1/2 Tbsp tomato paste
- 1/2 tsp salt

Instructions:

1. Place a Dutch oven over medium flame and heat the olive oil. Cook the chicken in it until

golden brown all over, then take it out of the Dutch oven and drain the oil. Put the chicken back in and sprinkle the onion on top.

2. In a bowl, mix together the broth, garlic, cinnamon, coriander, paprika, ginger, cumin, pepper, Splenda, cayenne, salt, and tomato past. Mix well and then pour this all over the chicken. Put the lid on the Dutch oven and set the heat on low.

3. Simmer for 30 minutes, then take off the lid and let simmer for an additional 10 minutes or until juices start to thicken. Serve with the juices spooned on top of each piece.

Low Carb Pasticchio

Makes: 3 servings

Ingredients:

- 1/2 small onion, chopped
- 1 small clove garlic, crushed
- 1/2 lb ground turkey
- 1/16 tsp ground nutmeg
- 1/3 tsp ground cinnamon
- 1/2 cup ricotta cheese
- 1/8 cup chopped fresh parsley
- 1/8 tsp salt
- 1/16 tsp pepper

For the sauce:

- 1 Tbsp butter
- 3/4 cup heavy cream
- 1/4 cup Parmesan cheese
- 1/4 tsp salt
- 1 cup cooked spaghetti squash

Instructions:

1. In a microwavable casserole, mix together the garlic and onion. Put the ground turkey on

top. Microwave, uncovered, at full power for 4 minutes. Stir to break up the ground turkey, then microwave everything for an additional 2 minutes and 30 seconds, or until the turkey becomes completely done.

2. With a fork, break up the ground turkey until completely crumbled and drain the fat from the casserole. Add the nutmeg and cinnamon and stir very well to combine. Microwave for 1 minute to let the flavors meld together. Spoon the turkey mixture into a mixing bowl.

3. In another bowl, mix together the parsley, ricotta cheese, salt, and pepper.

4. In a measuring cup, mix together the butter, cream, cheese, and sauce.

5. Grease the microwavable casserole with some oil or nonstick cooking spray. Spread out half of the spaghetti squash as the first layer, followed by half of the turkey mixture, then half of the ricotta mixture, and half the sauce. Repeat this procedure with the top layer as the sauce.

6. Microwave the dish for 5 minutes at full power or until heated through and bubbly. Set aside for a bit to cool down, then serve.

Greek Roasted Chicken

Makes: 2 to 3 servings

Ingredients:

- 2 lb chicken pieces

- 1/4 cup olive oil

- 1/8 cup lemon juice

- 1/4 tsp salt

- 1/8 tsp pepper

Instructions:

1. Wash the chicken pieces well and then pat them dry using paper towels.

2. In a bowl, mix together the olive oil, lemon juice, salt, and pepper. Put the chicken pieces in a resealable plastic bag and pour the marinade inside. Close the plastic bag and turn several times to coat.

3. Put the bag in the refrigerator to let the chicken marinate for 12 to 24 hours.

4. Take the chicken out of the bag and roast it in your oven for 375 degrees F for 45 minutes to 1 hour. You can also grill it until golden brown on both sides, about 10 to 15 minutes per side on medium flame. Serve with a salad.

Chapter 6 - Beef

Stir-Fried Ground Beef

Makes: 1 to 2 servings

Ingredients:

- 1 1/2 Tbsp dry sherry
- 1 Tbsp soy sauce
- 1 clove garlic, crushed
- 1/2 lb ground beef
- 1/4 cup coarsely chopped walnuts
- 1 cup frozen crosscut green beans, thawed
- 1 small onion, sliced
- 3/4 tsp grated fresh ginger
- Peanut oil for stir-frying

Instructions:

1. In a mixing bowl, mix together half of the measured sherry, 1/2 tablespoon soy sauce, and garlic. Put the ground beef into the mixture and mix well with clean hands.

2. Place a wok or heavy-duty skillet over high flame and heat a tablespoon or two of peanut oil. Add the walnuts and stir until crispy. Drain and set aside.

3. In the same wok, stir-fry the ground beef mixture until well done. Take the beef out of the wok and drain, then set aside.

4. Remove some of the fat and oil from the wok, and add about a tablespoonful of fresh peanut oil. On high flame, sauté the onion, ginger, and green beans until crisp and fork-tender.

5. Put the ground beef back into the wok and stir to combine. Add the rest of the sherry and sauce and stir well.

6. Sprinkle with toasted walnuts on top and serve, with or without whole grain brown or red rice.

Sesame Orange Beef

Makes: 2 servings

Ingredients:

- 1/2 lb beef chuck, sliced thin across the grain
- 1/3 cup white wine vinegar
- 1 tsp dark sesame oil
- 1 Tbsp Splenda
- 1/2 Tbsp soy sauce
- 1/2 tsp orange extract, divided
- 1 1/2 Tbsp peanut or canola oil
- 1/2 small onion, sliced
- 1/4 cup shredded carrots
- 1 cup frozen cross-cut green beans, thawed
- Xanthan or guar

Instructions:

1. Place the sliced beef inside a large resealable plastic bag. In a bowl, mix together the white wine vinegar, sesame oil, half of the orange extract, and Splenda. Pour the mixture into the plastic bag with the beef. Close the bag and flip several times to coat the beef with the mixture. Refrigerate for 12 to 24 hours.

2. Take the beef out of the fridge and transfer the marinade into a bowl. Add the remaining orange extract and the soy sauce. Stir and set aside.

3. Place a wok or heavy skillet over the highest possible setting and pour the oil. Once hot, put the beef inside and stir-fry until browned all over. Set aside on a plate.

4. Add more oil into the wok, then stir-fry the vegetables until fork-tender. Put the beef back in, as well as the marinade. Add a bit of xanthan or guar to thicken the sauce and stir until cooked through. Serve, preferably with a hot vegetable side dish.

No-noodle Lasagna

Makes: 2 servings

Ingredients:

- 1/2 lb ground beef
- 2 oz sliced mushrooms
- 1/2 cup low carb spaghetti sauce
- 1/2 cup ricotta cheese
- 1 small egg, beaten
- 3/4 cup shredded mozzarella cheese
- 1/4 tsp Italian seasoning
- 12 slices pepperoni

Instructions:

1. Preheat the oven to 350 degrees F.

2. Place a frying pan over medium heat and cook the ground beef until well done and browned. Drain the oil from the pan and add the mushrooms and spaghetti sauce to the ground beef. Simmer for 8 minutes.

3. In a bowl, combine the egg, Italian seasoning, ricotta, and 1/8 cup mozzarella. Combine well.

4. Lightly grease a small glass baking dish and spread the beef mixture in the bottom. Spread the egg and cheese mixture on top, then

arrange some of the pepperoni slices on top. Spread the rest of the mozzarella on top of the pepperoni slices, then arrange the remaining pepperoni slices on top.

5. Bake for about 15 to 20 minutes, or until bubbly. Slice and serve.

Bourbon Glazed Cajun Tenderloin

Makes: 4 servings

Ingredients:

- 1 1/2 lb center-cut beef tenderloin
- Extra virgin olive oil

For the marinade:

- 1/8 cup Worcestershire sauce
- 1 Tbsp Dijon mustard
- 1 Tbsp black strap molasses

For the meat rub:

- 1/2 Tbsp garlic powder
- 1/2 Tbsp cracked black pepper
- 1/2 Tbsp paprika
- 1 tsp salt
- 1/4 tsp cayenne red pepper

For the glaze:

- 1/8 cup Dijon mustard
- 1/8 cup bourbon
- 1 Tbsp black strap molasses

Instructions:

1. In a bowl, beat together all of the ingredients for the marinade.

2. Cut off the excess fat and silver skin from the beef tenderloin and place it in a resealable plastic bag. Pour the marinade in it and turn several times to coat. Refrigerate for at least 8 hours, preferably up to 24 hours.

3. To prepare the meat, take the meat out of the plastic bag and throw away the marinade. In a bowl, combine all of the ingredients for the meat rub. Pat the tenderloin dry with some paper towels, then vigorously apply the rub all over it. Set aside for half an hour to let the flavors penetrate the meat.

4. In another bowl, combine all of the glaze ingredients by whisking it all very well.

5. To start cooking the tenderloin, brush some extra virgin olive oil all over the meat. Heat up a skillet over medium-high flame and sear the tenderloin for 5 minutes per side.

6. Insert a meat thermometer in the thickest section of the tenderloin, then put it in a roasting pan. Cook for 50 minutes to an hour or until the meat thermometer reads 135 degrees. 10 minutes before the end of cooking time, brush the meat with the glaze mixture.

7. At the end of cooking time, take the tenderloin out of the oven and let stand for 10 minutes. The internal temperature will increase from 5 to 10 degrees, but make sure to serve it only if it reads at least 140 degrees F (which makes it medium-rare). Slice and serve.

Greek Shepherd's Pie

Makes: 2 servings

Ingredients:

- 1/2 lb ground beef
- 1 small onion, chopped
- 7 oz canned diced tomatoes, drained
- 7 oz canned crushed tomatoes or 4 oz canned tomato sauce
- 1 Tbsp minced garlic
- 2 to 3 tsp granulated Splenda
- 1/2 tsp oregano
- 1/2 tsp cinnamon or allspice
- 1/2 Tbsp Worcestershire sauce
- Salt
- Pepper
- 1 cup frozen cross-cut green beans, thawed
- 1/4 cup grated Parmesan

For the fauxtatoes:

- 2 cups fresh cauliflower
- 1 Tbsp butter
- 1/4 cup cream cheese with chives
- 1 small clove garlic, crushed

- Salt and pepper

Instructions:

1. Place a Dutch oven over medium-high heat and cook the ground beef until browned all over. Drain the fat, then add the chopped onion and cook until translucent.

2. Add the tomatoes, garlic, seasonings, green beans, and Splenda. Mix well and let simmer for 15 minutes. If it starts to dry up, just add a bit of water.

3. Meanwhile, make the fauxtatoes by steaming the cauliflower in a covered bowl of water in the microwave for 6 minutes, or until tender. Pop the cauliflower, cream cheese, garlic, and butter into a food processor and blend to a thick paste. Season with salt and pepper.

4. Spread the beef mixture into a small casserole and sprinkle the cheese on top. Add the mock fauxtatoes on top in an even layer.

5. Bake at 375 degrees F for 15 minutes or until the pie starts to brown and get bubbly. Take it out of the oven, sprinkle some more cheese on top, let it melt in the heat, then serve.

Chapter 7 - Pork

Italian Herb Pork Chops

Makes: 2 servings

Ingredients:

- 2 cloves garlic, crushed

- 1 tsp powdered sage, dried

- 2 pork chops, 1 inch thick

- 1 tsp powdered rosemary, dried

- Salt

- 1 Tbsp white wine

Instructions:

1. Rub the crushed garlic all over the pork chops.

2. Combine the powdered rosemary and sage in a small bowl and then sprinkle this all over the pork chop. Season the pork chops with salt.

3. Place a heavy skillet over low flame and place the pork chop in it. Pour just enough water in the skillet to cover the pork chop simmer and let simmer until the water completely evaporates.

4. After the water has evaporated, brown the chop on both sides carefully, as it will be more tender.

5. Take the pork chops out of the skillet and place them on a serving dish. Pour the dry white wine into the skillet and increase the temperature to medium-high. Mix the wine as you bring it to a boil. Boil for 1 minute, then pour this on top of the pork chops and serve.

Pork Chili

Makes: 2 servings

Ingredients:

- 1/3 cup chopped onion

- 2 cloves garlic, crushed

- 1 Tbsp olive oil

- 3/4 lb pork loin, boneless and cut into 1/2 inch cubes

- 1/2 green pepper, chopped

- 1 1/4 tsp chili powder

- 1/2 tsp ground cumin

- 1/2 cup chicken broth

- 1/8 cup picante sauce

- 2 chipotle chilies canned in adobo, minced

- 1 tsp adobo sauce from the chilies

- 1/8 cup pumpkin seed meal (pumpkin seeds ground in food processor)

- Salt

Instructions:

1. Place a heavy skillet or Dutch oven over medium flame and pour the olive oil. Heat it

up, then saute the garlic and onion until the onion becomes translucent.

2. Add the rest of the ingredients, except the pumpkin seed meal, into the mixture and cover. Let simmer for 45 minutes.

3. Add the pumpkin seed meal and stir to combine, then let simmer for an additional 10 minutes. Season with salt, and then serve.

Mu Shu Pork

Makes: 1 serving

Ingredients:

- 1 large egg, beaten

- 1/4 cup slivered mushrooms

- Peanut oil

- 4 oz boneless pork loin, sliced across the grain into matchstick-sized pieces

- 1/2 cup shredded napa cabbage

- 1/2 cup bean sprouts

- 2 scallions, sliced

- 1 1/2 Tbsp soy sauce

- 1 Tbsp dry sherry

- 2 low carb tortillas, warmed

For the hoisin sauce:

- 2 Tbsp soy sauce

- 1 Tbsp Splenda

- 1 Tbsp creamy natural peanut butter

- 1 tsp white vinegar

- 1 tsp toasted sesame oil

- 1 clove garlic, crushed

- 1/16 tsp Chinese Five Spice powder

Instructions:

1. To make the hoisin sauce, combine all of the ingredients for it in a food processor or a blender. Blend until smooth and thoroughly mixed. Store in a tight lid container.

2. Place a wok or heavy skillet over high flame and pour the peanut oil. Heat it up, then scramble the egg until half-cooked. Take it out of the wok and into a plate, then set aside.

3. Wipe the wok clean, removing traces of egg. Pour some more peanut oil and let it heat up. Stir-fry the pork in it until almost cooked. Add the scallions, cabbage, and sprouts. Stir-fry everything for 4 minutes, then add the half-cooked egg back in and stir to combine. Pour the soy sauce and sherry into the mixture and stir.

4. Transfer the pork mixture into a dish. To eat, spread a bit of hoisin sauce on the warmed tortilla and then spoon the pork mixture into it. Wrap it up and enjoy.

Spicy Pork Chops

Makes: 2 servings

Ingredients:

- 2 boneless pork chops, cut 1/2 inch thick
- 1/8 cup lime juice
- 1/2 Tbsp olive oil
- 1/2 Tbsp chili powder
- 1/2 tsp ground cumin
- 1/2 tsp ground cinnamon
- 1/4 tsp hot pepper sauce
- 1/8 tsp salt
- 1 clove garlic, minced

Instructions:

1. Trip the pork chops and put them in a bowl. In a smaller bowl, mix together the olive oil, lime juice, chili powder, cinnamon, cumin, garlic, hot pepper sauce, and salt. Pour the mixture all over the pork chops and turn to coat.

2. Cover the pork chops and place them in the refrigerator for 6 to 12 hours, turning the chops every time you remember to do so.

3. Preheat the charcoal grill and drain the pork chops. Grill them for 10 minutes, turning once,

or until the juices run clear and the internal temperature is at 160 degrees F. Serve.

Pork Chops in Cream Sauce Topped with Seasoned Goat Cheese

Makes: 2 servings

Ingredients:

- 2 pork chops, boneless
- 1/2 Tbsp olive oil
- 1 1/2 Tbsp butter
- 1/2 shallot, chopped
- 1 clove garlic, chopped
- 3 mushrooms, sliced
- 1 1/2 Tbsp sherry
- 1/2 Tbsp fresh thyme, chopped
- 1/2 Tbsp fresh oregano, chopped
- 1/2 tsp fresh rosemary, finely chopped
- 1/2 cup heavy cream
- 4 oz goat cheese
- 1 small clove garlic, chopped fine
- 1/2 tsp fresh thyme, chopped
- 1/2 tsp fresh oregano, chopped
- Salt
- Pepper

Instructions:

1. Season the pork chops with salt and pepper.

2. Place a heavy skillet over medium flame and cook the pork chops for 4 minutes per side or until browned. Set aside on a plate.

3. Drain the oil from the pan and melt the butter in it over medium flame. Sauté the shallot and 1 clove of garlic for 1 minute then add the mushrooms and season with some salt and pepper. Cook for 2 minutes until soft.

4. Pour the sherry into the mushroom mixture and add the first batch of herbs. Sauté and bring to a boil until sherry is reduced. Add the cream and stir to mix.

5. Put the pork chops back into the skillet with the sauce. Turn to coat and let simmer for 5 minutes.

6. Meanwhile, combine the garlic, the remaining herbs, and goat cheese in a small bowl.

7. Take the pork chops and place them on a serving plate. Sprinkle the goat cheese mixture on top and then drizzle the cream sauce all over everything. Serve immediately.

Chapter 8 - Seafood

Orange Swordfish Steaks with Almonds

Makes: 1 to 2 servings

Ingredients:

- 10 oz swordfish steak

- 1 Tbsp olive oil

- 1/3 tsp orange extract

- 1 tsp Splenda

- 1/8 cup lemon juice

- 1 Tbsp butter

- 1 Tbsp slivered almonds

Instructions:

1. In a bowl, mix together the olive oil, lemon juice, orange extract, and Splenda. Place the swordfish steak in a resealable plastic bag, and pour the mixture in with it.

2. Seal the bag and turn the bag twice to coat the fish in the mixture. Put it in the fridge and let it marinate for 1 hour, turning sit several times.

3. Grease a nonstick skillet with half of the butter. Melt over low flame and then place the

swordfish steak on top. Pour the marinade into a bowl. Cook one side of the swordfish steak for 5 minutes, then flip over carefully and cook the other side for 5 minutes as well.

4. In a smaller skillet over medium flame, melt the remaining amount of butter and add the almonds. Stir frequently in the butter until golden. Remove from heat and set aside.

5. After the swordfish steak is cooked, pour the marinade into the pan and let it simmer for 2 minutes, turning once. Transfer to a serving plate and drizzle the sauce on top. Sprinkle the almonds on top and serve.

Tilapia with Vegetables

Makes: 2 servings

Ingredients:

- 1 1/2 Tbsp olive oil
- 1/2 cup yellow bell pepper, sliced into thin strips
- 1/2 cup red bell pepper, sliced into thin strips
- 3/4 cup zucchini, sliced into matchstick strips
- 3/4 cups yellow squash, sliced into matchstick strips
- 1/2 cup sweet red onion, sliced thinly
- 1/2 lb tilapia fillets
- 1 small clove garlic, crushed
- Salt
- Pepper
- 1/8 tsp guar or xanthan
- Lemon wedges, for serving

Instructions:

1. Season the tilapia fillets with a bit of salt and pepper.

2. Place a heavy-duty skillet over medium-high flame and heat the olive oil. Saute the onion, garlic, peppers, zucchini, and squash for 2 minutes.

3. Put the tilapia fillets on top of the vegetables in the skillet. Cover, then reduce heat to medium-low and let it steam up for about 8 minutes, or until the tilapia is done.

4. Carefully place the tilapia fillets onto a serving platter using a spatula. Pile the vegetables on top of the fillets using a slotted spoon.

5. Pour the liquids from the skillet into a blender or food processor and add the guar or xanthan. Blend until thickened, then drizzle the sauce on top of the vegetables and fillets. Serve with lemon wedges, if desired.

Salmon Stuffed with Cilantro, Lime, Scallions, and Anaheim Peppers

Makes: 6 servings

Ingredients:

- Half a salmon, about 3 lbs, cleaned and gutted
- 1/2 lime, sliced paper-thin
- 1/2 Anaheim chili pepper, sliced into matchstick thin strips
- 1 scallion, sliced thin lengthwise
- 1/2 bunch cilantro, chopped
- 1 Tbsp olive oil

Instructions:

1. Preheat the oven to 350 degrees F. Generously grease a roasting pan with nonstick cooking spray.

2. Place the salmon on the prepared roasting pan. Stuff it with the lime, Anaheim chili pepper, scallion, and cilantro. Make sure to distribute everything as evenly as possible.

3. With a heavy thread and a needle, sew up the fish to prevent the stuffing from coming out during the cooking process. Rub the olive oil all over the fish.

4. Bake for 30 minutes. Attach a thermometer in the thickest part of the fish to check for readiness. It will be ready to eat once the thermometer reads 135 to 140 degrees F.

5. Slice the fish and serve with the stuffing.

Shrimp and Artichoke Cauliflower Risotto

Makes: 2 servings

Ingredients:

- 1/4 head cauliflower, shredded
- 1/4 cup chopped onion
- 2 cloves garlic
- 1/2 Tbsp dried or 1/8 cup chopped fresh basil
- 1/2 Tbsp olive oil
- 1/2 tsp salt
- 1/2 Tbsp lemon juice
- 1/4 tsp pepper
- 7 oz canned artichoke hearts, drained and chopped
- 1/2 tsp Creole seasoning
- 1/4 lb small shrimp
- 1/4 cup heavy cream
- 2 scallions, sliced
- 1/3 cup grated Parmesan cheese
- Xanthan or guar

Instructions:

1. Place the cauliflower inside a microwavable casserole that has a lid. Pour a bit of water in it, cover, and microwave for 4 minutes on high.

2. Place a large skillet over medium-low flame and heat the olive oil in it. Sauté the garlic and onion for about 3 minutes.

3. Take out the cauliflower from the microwave and drain it, then throw it into the skillet with the garlic and onions. Add the lemon juice, basil, salt, pepper, Creole seasoning, shrimp, cream, and artichoke hearts. Mix very well and let simmer for 2 minutes to let the flavors combine well.

4. Add the scallions and Parmesan cheese and stir. Add a bit of xanthan or guar to thicken the sauce, then remove from the heat and transfer into a serving dish.

Scallops on Spinach with Walnut Sauce

Makes: 2 servings

Ingredients:

- 6 oz large sea scallops

- 1/2 lb turkey bacon

- 1/2 lb spinach

- Peanut oil

For the walnut sauce:

- 1 cup water

- 1 Tbsp lemon juice

- 1/8 cup chopped walnuts

- 1/2 tsp lemon rind, grated

- 2 Tbsp extra virgin olive oil

- 1/4 tsp salt

- 1/4 tsp black pepper, freshly ground

Instructions:

1. Put the water in a saucepan over medium flame and bring to a boil. Add the walnuts and boil for 30 seconds. Drain and put the walnuts in a bowl. Add the olive oil, lemon juice, lemon rind, salt, pepper, and olive oil. Mix well and set aside.

2. Slice the turkey bacon pieces in half and wrap each scallop with a piece of turkey bacon. Put the wrapped scallops onto a skewer and baste with some peanut oil.

3. Wash the spinach leaves well, then place over high heat and cook until wilted. Broil the scallops for 5 minutes per side, basting every now and then.

4. Arrange the cooked spinach on a serving platter and place the broiled scallops on top. Drizzle the walnut sauce all over everything, and then serve.

Chapter 9 - Hot Vegetables

Turnips Au Gratin

Makes: 3 servings

Ingredients:

- 1 lb turnips, peeled and sliced thinly

- 1/2 cup heavy cream

- 1/2 cup half-and-half

- 1 tsp prepared horseradish

- 1 1/2 cups shredded sharp Cheddar cheese

- 1/8 tsp ground nutmeg

- 1/2 small onion, sliced

- Salt

- Pepper

Instructions:

1. Preheat the oven to 350 degrees F.

2. Steam the turnips until fork tender.

3. In a saucepan, mix together the half-and-half and heavy cream and stir over the lowest possible heat setting. Bring to a simmer, then add two-thirds of the measured Cheddar cheese. Stir until cheese becomes completely

melted. Add the nutmeg and horseradish and stir well. Remove from heat.

4. Lightly grease a small glass baking dish, then place a third of the turnips into it. Place some of the sliced onion on top. Add another third of the turnips and then the onions, and then top with the rest of the turnips. Pour the cheese mixture on top of everything and sprinkle the remaining Cheddar cheese on top. Bake for half an hour or until golden, then serve.

Holiday Green Bean Casserole

Makes: 3 servings

Ingredients:

- 1 small onion
- 1/8 tsp salt
- 1/8 cup rice protein powder or low carb bake mix
- 1/8 tsp paprika
- 2 cups frozen green beans, cut style
- 2 oz canned mushrooms
- 1 Tbsp minced onion
- 1/2 Tbsp butter
- 1/2 cup heavy cream
- 1/4 tsp chicken or beef bouillon concentrate
- 1/4 tsp Worcestershire sauce
- 1/2 tsp soy sauce
- Salt
- Pepper
- 1/4 tsp xanthan or guar
- Oil for frying

Instructions:

1. Slice the onion thinly and separate the rings. In a bowl, combine the protein powder or bake mix, paprika, and salt. Coat the onion rings in the flour mixture. You can do this by putting the flour in a paper bag and then adding the onion rings a few at a time into it, then shake.

2. Place a heavy skillet over medium flame and heat about a quarter of an inch high of oil in it. Fry the flour coated onion rings, flipping only once, until golden brown and crispy. Drain on paper towels.

3. Steam the green beans. You can do this by putting them in a microwavable bowl and microwaving them on high for 5 minutes with a bowl of water in the microwave with them.

4. Drain and reserve the mushroom liquids from the can. Put a skillet over low-medium flame and melt the butter, Sauté the minced onion and mushrooms until onion becomes soft and translucent. Add the cream, the mushroom liquids, Worcestershire sauce, soy sauce, and the bouillon concentrate. Stir well, then season with some salt and pepper.

5. Transfer the mixture into a blender and add the xanthan or guar. Blend until thickened, but make sure that the mushrooms do not become pureed.

6. Lightly grease a half quart casserole dish. Preheat the oven to 350 degrees F.

7. Drain your steamed green beans and put them in the prepared casserole dish. Pour the mushroom mixture into it and stir in about half of the fried onion rings. Bake for 20 minutes, then sprinkle the remaining fried onions on top and bake for an additional 3 minutes. Serve.

Mushroom and Spinach Casserole

Makes: 2 to 3 servings

Ingredients:

- 2 Tbsp butter

- 1/2 lb fresh mushrooms, sliced

- 1/4 cup parsley or any other mixed herbs of your choice

- 1/8 cup chopped onion

- 5 oz frozen chopped spinach, thawed and drained well

- 1/2 cup grated Swiss cheese or any other cheese of your choice

- 1/6 cup heavy cream

- 1 medium egg

- 1 egg yolk

- Parmesan cheese, as topping

Instructions:

1. Preheat the oven to 325 degrees F. Lightly grease a casserole dish with nonstick cooking spray or oil.

2. Place a skillet over medium flame and melt about half a tablespoon of butter in it. Saute the sliced mushrooms and let all the liquid evaporate from them. Set aside in a bowl.

3. Using the same skillet, melt another half tablespoon of butter and saute the onion until translucent and tender. Add the herbs and cook until fragrant, then transfer this mixture into the bowl with the mushrooms.

4. Put the spinach into the mushroom mixture and combine thoroughly. Set aside to cool to room temperature, then add the cheese and mix well. Transfer into the prepared casserole dish.

5. In another dish, beat together the egg, egg yolk, and cream. Spread this mixture on top of the mixed vegetables and sprinkle the Parmesan cheese on top.

6. Bake for about 25 minutes or until the cheese is melted and bubbly. Serve.

Chili Garlic Lime Pumpkin

Makes: 4 servings

Ingredients:

- 1 lb pumpkin
- 1 Tbsp butter
- 1/2 Tbsp coconut oil
- 1/4 cup shelled pumpkin seeds
- 1 tsp lime juice
- 1/2 tsp chili garlic paste

Instructions:

1. Scoop out the pumpkin seeds and peel off the hard rind. Slice the pumpkin flesh into about 1/4 inch thick pieces.

2. Combine the coconut oil and butter in a heavy skillet and place it over medium flame. Melt and spread all over the base of the pan. Place the pieces of pumpkin in the pan and sauté until tender and lightly golden all over. Set aside and cover to keep warm.

3. Place a dry skillet over medium-high flame and toast the shelled pumpkin seeds for about 3 minutes or until they start to swell. Take them off the heat and set aside.

4. Combine the chili garlic paste and lime juice in a bowl. Put the pumpkin pieces back into the

skillet and add the chili garlic paste and lime juice mixture. Stir to coat all of the pieces.

5. Spoon the pumpkin pieces on a plate and spoon the toasted pumpkin seeds on top. Serve immediately.

Kolokythia Krokettes

Makes: 3 servings

Ingredients:

- 2 small zucchini, grated
- 1/2 tsp salt
- 2 eggs
- 1/2 cup crumbled feta
- 1/4 medium onion, finely diced
- 1/2 tsp dried oregano
- 1/16 tsp pepper
- 1 1/2 Tbsp rice protein powder or soy powder
- Butter

Instructions:

1. In a mixing bowl, toss the grated zucchini with the salt and set aside for at least an hour. Squeeze out the liquid and set aside.

2. In another bowl, combine the oregano, eggs, feta, soy powder, onion, and pepper. Mix well.

3. Grease a heavy-duty skillet and melt a tablespoonful of butter over medium flame. Put some of the batter into the skillet and fry, turning only once. Cook the rest of the batch and pile on a plate, then serve.

Chapter 10 - Desserts

Peanut Butter Brownies

Makes: 8 brownies

Ingredients:

- 2 1/2 Tbsp butter, melted
- 1/8 cup unsweetened baking cocoa
- 1 egg
- 1/8 cup water
- 1/8 cup heavy cream
- 1/8 cup Splenda
- 1/2 tsp vanilla extract
- 1/2 tsp liquid saccharine
- 1/3 cup vanilla-flavored whey protein powder
- 1 Tbsp oat flour
- 1/2 Tbsp baking powder

For the peanut butter topping:

- 1/8 cup natural peanut butter
- 1 Tbsp Splenda
- 1 1/2 Tbsp butter
- 1 small egg

- 1/2 Tbsp vanilla-flavored whey protein powder

Instructions:

1. Preheat the oven to 350 degrees F.

2. Combine the melted butter, cocoa, cream, egg, water, Splenda, liquid saccharine, and vanilla extract. Add the oat flour, baking powder, and protein powder, then mix well.

3. Lightly grease a baking pan, then transfer the batter into it.

4. In a bowl, combine the peanut butter topping ingredients very well, then spread this all over the top of the brownie batter.

5. Bake for 12 to 15 minutes. Set aside to cool for a bit, then cut and serve.

Almond Cookies

Makes: 18 big cookies

Ingredients:

- 1/2 cup butter, at room temperature

- 1 small egg, beaten

- 1/2 cup Splenda

- 1/2 cup smooth almond butter

- 1/4 tsp baking soda

- 1/4 tsp salt

- 3/4 cup vanilla-flavored whey protein powder

- 1 Tbsp water

- 15 whole, shelled almonds

Instructions:

1. Preheat the oven to 375 degrees F. Grease a cookie sheet.

2. Put the butter in a mixing bowl and beat with an electric mixer until fluffy, then add the Splenda and beat to mix. Add the egg, almond butter, baking soda, and salt and beat until smooth. Add the protein powder gradually as you beat, followed by the water. Mix everything very well.

3. Form the cookies by scooping out two tablespoons of dough and form each into a ball. Place the balls on the prepared cookie sheet and push an almond in the center of each.

4. Bake for 10 minutes or until cookies start to become brown at the edges. Set aside to cool for a bit, then serve.

Dark Chocolate Cheesecake

Makes: 6 servings

Ingredients:

For the hazelnut crust:

- 3/4 cup hazelnuts
- 1/6 cup vanilla-flavored whey protein powder
- 2 Tbsp melted butter

For the bottom layer:

- 3 oz sugar-free dark chocolate bars
- 1/8 cup heavy cream

For the filling:

- 16 oz cream cheese, softened
- 1/3 cup Splenda
- 1/3 cup sour cream
- 2 eggs
- 1/2 Tbsp vanilla extract
- 1 Tbsp water
- 1 Tbsp Splenda
- 1/2 tsp instant coffee crystals
- A few drops of vanilla extract
- 1/2 tsp vodka

Instructions:

1. Make the hazelnut crust first. Preheat the oven to 350 degrees F.

2. Attach the S blade into the food processor and pulse the hazelnuts to a medium-fine ground. Add the butter and protein powder and pulse to mix.

3. Spray a spring form pan with nonstick cooking spray and press the hazelnut mixture evenly and firmly into it. Cover the seam around the bottom part of the spring form pan by pressing the mixture over it.

4. Put the pan on the lowest rack of the oven and bake for 12 minutes or until lightly browned. Take it out and set it aside.

5. Combine the tablespoon of Splenda with tablespoon of water, half teaspoon coffee crystals, vanilla extract, and vodka in a liquid container with a lid. Cover and shake well. Set aside.

6. Preheat the oven to 325 degrees F.

7. Using a double boiler or heat diffuser, melt the chocolate bars, then add the cream and mix well. Pour the mixture over the crust and spread it out evenly.

8. In a bowl, beat the cream cheese with an electric mixture until smooth. Add the sour cream and Splenda and beat well. Add the eggs

and vanilla and mix well. Add the vodka mixture, then mix very well.

9. Pour the filling over the chocolate-layered crust. Fill a pie pan with some water and put it in the oven. On the rack above this, place the unbaked cheesecake. Bake for 45 minutes, then set aside to cool on a wire rack.

10. Chill before slicing and serving.

Coconut Shortbread

Makes: 24 cookies

Ingredients:

- 1/4 cup butter, at room temperature

- 1 1/2 Tbsp Splenda

- 1/4 cup coconut oil

- 3/4 cup vanilla-flavored whey protein powder

- 1/2 cup finely shredded, unsweetened coconut

- 1 Tbsp water

Instructions:

1. Preheat the oven to 375 degrees F. Line a jelly roll pan using parchment paper.

2. In a mixing bowl, combine the butter, Splenda, and coconut oil using an electric mixer. Beat until creamy, then add the protein powder, coconut, and water and beat until thoroughly combined.

3. Transfer the dough into the prepared jelly roll pan and put another sheet of parchment paper on top. Press the dough out to create a thin sheet. Score the dough using a sharp knife or a pizza cutter into small rectangles.

4. Bake for 7 minutes or until pale brown, and then set aside to cool on a rack. Break apart and serve.

Mocha Custard

Makes: 2 servings

Ingredients:

- 1/2 cup boiling water

- 1/2 oz unsweetened baking chocolate

- 1/2 tsp instant coffee crystals

- 2 small eggs

- 1/2 cup heavy cream

- 1/6 cup Splenda

- Salt

Instructions:

1. Preheat the oven to 300 degrees F.

2. Combine the chocolate and boiling water in a blender and let it stand for about 5 minutes. Then add the eggs, coffee crystals, Splenda, and heavy cream. Add a light dash of salt and blend for 1 minute.

3. Lightly grease a half-quart baking dish and transfer the mocha mixture into it. Put the baking fish in a big pan filled with hot water and place it in the oven. Bake for 50 minutes.

4. Set aside to cool first, and then chill for at least 1 hour before you serve.

Conclusion

Thank you again for buying this book!

I hope this book was able to help you lose weight and adapt a healthier lifestyle by preparing healthy and delicious food everyday.

The next step is to continue improving your lifestyle choices and add more delectable low carb recipes to your collection.

Finally, if you enjoyed this book, please take the time to share your thoughts and post a review on Amazon. It'd be greatly appreciated!

Thank you and good luck!

Made in the USA
Middletown, DE
16 January 2015